THE
Menopause
Diet

The Feel-Good,
Lose-Weight Plan for the
Menopausal Woman

D0062179

ALLAN N. SPREEN, M.D., C.N.C.

WOODLAND PUBLISHING
Pleasant Grove, Utah

My thanks to Hi Health manager Mona Wooten for suggesting this booklet and to my sister Cathy for inspiration and encouragement.

© 1999
Woodland Publishing
P.O. Box 160
Pleasant Grove, Utah
84062

CONTENTS

INTRODUCTION

Everything sort of hits at once. You're in the neighborhood of fifty (a fun milestone of its own); controlling your weight is now tougher (however tough it ever was); you feel irritable (not your fault); and, (just for grins) you have hot flashes. It just isn't fair (and it makes me appreciate being a guy).

Everyone knows that menopause is a time of hormonal changes. There's no news there, and also nothing at all in that information to help you lose weight. The ending of a woman's ovulatory cycles can be responsible for all sorts of miseries for many women, though for some there are basically no symptoms at all.

This is not a text book on either menopause or the conventional hormone therapies for it. You can get a whole bunch of big, technical volumes for that. Let's keep it as simple as possible. Our purpose is to work with the realities of menopause while trying to accomplish two things: 1) how to lose weight when stuck within the age of menopause; and 2) how to feel better while trying to handle the hassles of menopause.

The second factor is intimately linked to the first. If you feel like a lump of hot, crabby, death-warmed-over, you won't have the drive to work on trimming down. Plus, that lousy feeling may be a symptom of not only decreasing estrogen, but also decreasing thyroid hormone, which can have a very direct impact on weight loss.

It will be necessary, however, to understand just a little about the processes at work in a woman's body (not that any guy could ever really do that) to better utilize the tricks we wish to employ for our "double-barreled" purpose. Double-barreled is an appropriate image, because this plan nearly always ends up necessarily being a shotgun approach, at least to some degree. Weight loss, for most, is difficult in the first place, without the additional physical and emotional stresses of menopause. For others, a trim figure has never been a problem. Then menopause hits, and all of a sudden the victim looks in the mirror and can't recognize the body looking back.

In terms of losing weight, there are things you can do, and those efforts do not include counting either calories or fat grams. And I know, I know, you've heard that before. But bear with me. We need a little introduction so I have a chance to adequately defend myself (and to adequately help you lose weight).

FOOD ATTITUDES

Most people assume that a calorie is a calorie. Both common sense and scientific reality tell us that's true, and in a test tube, yes, all calories are equal. The problem, however, is the human body throws some curve balls into the equation, and it's not the test tube's measurements we're trying to change.

You may have seen it yourself. You cut out 3,500 calories over some period of time and, with no other changes, you lose a pound. You try it for the second pound, and you lose less than a pound. You try it for the fifth pound, and you lose maybe half a pound, maybe even less. What's going on here? This is true for nonmenopausal women (and men) as well. It's not just the famous explanation of "water weight" either (though at times there is something to that).

Your metabolism slows down when it realizes that you have eaten less than it was used to. It must assume, over many generations of reinforcement, that you are having trouble getting food, so the defense mechanisms take over to protect you from potentially starving. It makes you tired or lowers your body's heat-generating apparatus to conserve energy (calories). Just what a woman needs during her fifties—less energy to do the things she wants or needs to do! There are games you can play, but counting calories is not the best one for this purpose.

Counting fat grams is an even poorer idea for menopausal women. The lack of essential fatty acids in a conventional low-fat routine can wreak even more havoc on a woman's hormones right when she's having more trouble with them than she may have ever had since she started having periods. Even saturated fats are worth having around.

What's worse, low-fat diets are nearly always high in carbohydrates. There just isn't that much else to eat if you decide to cut out the fat; there is protein, and there are carbohydrates (carbs), and that's it. The taste that you give up with a low-fat diet is compensated for by using carbohydrates, and refined carbohydrates at that. We are told that fat has more calories per gram than carbohydrate, and though technically it's true, it is more difficult to eat as many grams of fat than grams of refined, simple carbohydrates. Fat shuts off your appetite; carbs stimulate it. We'll discuss this more later, but keep in mind that this point merits a dieter's consideration.

SUPPLEMENTATION

There is a good chance that the food you eat is not enough to fulfill your health needs, no matter how well you select it. With bad soil, bad water, fast foods, synthetic additives, food refining and processing, personal genetic imperfections, constant environmental and emotional stresses, medications, and just the inevitable stress of aging, there is little chance that what you eat will be adequate. Just having good, fresh food hang around too long makes it less than perfect.

My approach to treating menopause includes, of course, the food you eat, but of necessity there must be more. Nutritional/dietary supplements almost certainly will be necessary. Some may be more effective in your personal situation, some less. You need to evaluate each supplemental "piece," then decide if it fits into the puzzle that is you. Some pieces help other pieces fit better, and some may be totally exclusive, but necessary to fit your biochemical individuality.

There are supplements that have a long history of assisting women in their efforts to comfortably enjoy their "golden years." Whether your needs are greater than normal, your intake is less, or your utilization is poor, a trial of selected nutrients can make a significant difference. Some may even be the answer to assuring that all the other nutrients are adequately absorbed. I have seen this be the answer in several areas of the quest for health, and it's worth considering in yours.

Some specific herbs can make the process of menopause bearable, and in some cases can mean the difference between feeling enthusiastic about real improvement and total complacency about how you look or feel. Hormonal involvement of your thyroid is also possible, in addition to the obvious importance of your ovaries. I strongly believe that even normal blood tests for thyroid function may not be sensitive enough to rule out the possibility that a sub-clinically weak thyroid may be causing you to feel worse than you should and adversely affecting your ability to lose weight.

To help you put together this puzzle, I recommend that you find a health-care practitioner willing to consider alternatives to synthetic hormones or other drugs for your problem. Either way, you should have a professional monitor your efforts.

My approach to menopause is based in the idea that menopause is a sign of slowing down of several processes, not just estrogen. Therefore we want to enhance more than just one process, particularly as they pertain to the digestion and absorption of food, energy-utilization, hormone levels, and even mood. If you feel better emotionally you'll be better able to aggressively pursue other aspects of attaining good health.

The water is muddied by the fact that there is no perfect diet for everyone; otherwise there would only be one diet, and everyone would use it. As you may have noticed, such is not the case. Despite the fact that developing one's own diet will require some effort, it does not have to be too complicated.

To resolve the diet dilemma, we make this plan flexible. We have to do this, or we'd be skirting the issue using a single-shot idea that, if it didn't work, would leave you out in the cold (or hot, in your case). Plus, if your situation is more involved with hot flashes than weight control problems, or vice versa, you can emphasize the plan areas that best suit your personal needs. Everyone is different.

In the next sections of this book, we will go through the steps by which you can design the program that best—or most easily—controls your menopausal symptoms *and* your ability to lose weight during the menopausal period. Once you find what parts of the regimen work for you, you'll be well on your way to solving the problem. Best of luck, and good health!

Menopause and Diet

Unfortunately, there need to be a few dietary rules for your success. However, it will not be necessary, in my opinion, for you to weigh portions, count calories, or measure fat grams. In fact, you might be shocked if you did, in this plan, so don't. One bit of bad news is that the food part of this plan is politically incorrect, so your friends may tell you you're crazy to try it. You can find out whether these ideas make you gain or lose in plenty of time to trash the idea if it isn't working. (I don't think you'll find that to be the case.)

In short, the low fat mindset is out the window, and carbohydrates, especially the refined ones, are generally considered the guys worthy of considerable "fear." As we've mentioned, most low-fat regimens are usually high in carbohydrate content. Other than protein, there just isn't that much else to eat. This gives the menopausal woman not just one stress to deal with, but a double-whammy. Carbohydrates (sugars, fruits, starches, grains, flours, etc.) require insulin for their metabolism. As soon as you eat them, you get an increase in blood sugar, rapidly followed by a slug of insulin from the pancreas to move that sugar into either muscle cells, if you burn it all, or into fat cells if you don't (fun thought).

These days, most carbohydrates are highly refined. The sugar has had all the vitamins, minerals, phytonutrients and fiber removed, so it has little resemblance to the original sugarcane or sugar beet. In addition, flour used in bread products has had nearly all its fiber and most of its nutrients removed, while the amount of synthetic "enrichment" that is sprinkled back is negligible. This "enrichment" process has no fiber and no minerals at all, and the few vitamins aren't worth mentioning, but it does do a pretty good job of selling bread.[1]

Our goal is to subject your system to the lowest carbohydrate stress possible. This is important because carbohydrates *require* insulin to be metabolized, while proteins and fats don't. Whenever you get a surge of insulin (after a carbohydrate-rich meal), you *completely* shut down any fat-burning processes going on in your body.[2] If your dietary intake is comprised predominantly of refined carbohydrates (which it is if you're a normal American), the result is even worse.

Though this "plan" has rules, they are general enough and flexible enough to give all menopausal women a good shot at having them work. As you may have guessed, you won't get specific daily diet plans, or a strict regimen of individual meals. However, there is an excellent chance you won't need them. If you just must have such rigid guidelines, I'll tell you where you can easily acquire them.

With guidelines on eating proteins, fats, and carbohydrates, and a bit of education about what foods actually are proteins, fats, and good carbohydrates, you'll have a dietary regimen that allows you to eat anywhere, anytime, and still remain within the plan's boundaries. Once you have found a general routine that best suits you, there are several books listed in the section on "Nutrient Density" that include recipes and meals to help you keep this routine.

The Plan

Here's the plan: For the first week you eat foods that allow basically no carbohydrate intake at all (mmm, fun week). This is when you learn the most about how your body has been responding to carbohydrates. You'll probably lose a fair amount of weight during that period, but you may have no desire to continue eating that way. You also may feel worse at first, and better later. That's common, but not universal.

A week of eating this way usually puts most people into a fat-burning biochemical state called "ketosis," not to be confused with "ketoacidosis," (which is quite a bit different and dangerous). During ketosis the body preferentially burns fat for energy.[3] By avoiding carbohydrates altogether, a great deal may be learned about how the body can respond to stresses like menopause when fats are the primary energy source. This dietary method was made famous many years ago by Robert Atkins, M.D., in his book *The Atkins Diet Revolution*. His work with thousands of patients proved the efficacy of such eating techniques.

During the ketosis process, you may notice a sweetish breath, and you may even have a change in body odor as you start burning fat that hasn't been burned before. Other symptoms may occur: your tongue may become coated as toxins are liberated from fat stores, your energy may increase or decrease, you could have mild aching, or you may even experience mood elevation. (The state of ketosis can be detected by the use of "ketostix," available at most pharmacies.)

After the first week you begin adding carbohydrates (good carbohydrates, that is) into your diet. You do this by introducing unrefined carbs that also tend to be low on a scale called the *glycemic index* (see table, p. 27). These are sugars and starches that are thought to minimally stress the pancreas (your insulin maker) and cause a small release of insulin into the bloodstream. You can then add more carbohydratess until you find a balance point between the optimum amounts and types of carbohydrates you can tolerate, and continued weight loss, symptom relief, or both. However, whichever carbohydrates you decide to consume, they need to remain as unrefined as absolutely possible.

Unfortunately, there's a small problem with the glycemic index. I am not convinced that the final verdict is in concerning the absolute accuracy of this list. Different versions have different rankings and, far more important, some foods with minimal nutritional value are ranked higher on the list, while some wholesome ones are represented as "worse." That's why we won't use the index as a hard and fast guide. It will give us some good guidance, however, and that's what we need.

You'll be able to cheat without major feelings of guilt. However, if you cheat too far from the guidelines (after the first week or so), you'll feel worse physically, and that tends to reinforce compliance. Most people get very familiar with the foods that work for them and the foods that don't. Everyone's biochemistry is different, so it's silly to make too many black-and-white rules that may not apply to you. We'll keep such rules to a minimum—life's tough enough.

NUTRIENT DENSITY

The main factor we seek is "nutrient density," for which there is no official list. This involves the application of common sense combined with some general guidelines. It makes the diet more workable, and therefore easier to implement as a permanent change in lifestyle.

The concept of nutrient density allows us to analyze any food, anywhere, and evaluate its chances of helping us improve or worsen our health. Any food in nature contains within itself all the nutrients required for the assimilation of that food (assuming it was grown in a wholesome setting with as few man-made additives as possible). In the case of sweet foods, this means things like magnesium, vitamins B_1 and B_6, chromium, fiber, and many other things. If the food doesn't supply it, the body will take from body stores to get it. If your body doesn't happen to have adequate stores, you get sick.

The point is that as soon as a food is processed in any way, it loses some of its nutrient density. Whether it be by freezing, boiling, frying, gassing, irradiating, coloring, flavor-enhancing, or preserving, food becomes less than it was. Plus, there are various things done to our food as it grows—hormones, pesticides, weed killers, antibiotics, synthetic fertilizers—that contribute to this lessening. With my approach, we will endeavor to stick with nutrient-dense foods so the body has the best chance to maximize the process of feeling better and normalizing weight. Organic foods from an established, reputable organic rating system (not the Department of Agriculture) are the best.

Books that contain excellent recipes for these types of meals include Robert Atkins' *The Diet Revolution* and *The New Diet Revolution*; *The Zone Diet*, by Barry Sears; *40-30-30 Fat Burning Nutrition*, by Daoust and Daoust; and *The Carbohydrate Addict's Diet*, by Heller and Heller. Of course there are others; simply look for recipes that emphasize lower carbohydrate ratios.

A really magnificent book, loaded not only with wonderful recipes but also an incredible education, is *Nourishing Traditions*, by Sally Fallon. This work shows in no uncertain terms that the modern high-carbohydrate, low-fat diets have never been the way man was meant to eat. However many carbohydrates you decide to include in your diet (after the first week), remember this caveat: Whatever carbohydrates you eat should be *as unrefined as possible*. I can't stress this enough. We all know you're going to cheat sometime. There will come those moments when a hot fudge sundae with all the trimmings, or even just a big fat yeast roll, is a mandatory food item. The point is, be aware that you are cheating, and be on the lookout for a possible worsening of your symptoms. You're trying to stress your body as little as possible, and eating refined carbohydrate is the best way to do the exact opposite, all low-fat lore to the contrary.[4]

Although a fair amount of fat is allowed in this approach, some types of fat need to be avoided. We'll try to steer clear of them, as they are just another burden that can chemically mess up an already burdened menopausal system. The final section of this booklet lists foods in each category and rankings in the Glycemic Index, which uses glucose at a rank of 100 as the indicator around which other foods are compared. For now, here are some basics, necessary for the beginner, so we all know we're communicating on the same wavelength.

CARBOHYDRATES

Carbohydrates are the sugars and starches. They include fruits, vegetables, caloric sweeteners like honey and maple syrup, flours, cereals, breads, pastas, and other starches. As I've said, some carbs are worse than others. These include both the refined and high glycemic-index types. Most of the refined carbs have a high glycemic index, but this is not always the case. How much you add back into your diet depends on your personal biochemistry and desire to handle symptoms and weight. These are the foods that can make the most trouble in the least amount of time.

Refining is processing done by the food industry in order to increase the shelf life of certain foods. By removing fiber and nutrients, foods can be made to last longer on shelves before going bad. The important parts of the food can also be turned into animal chows, with the useless portions turned into foods like refined breakfast cereals that we humans are dumb enough to eat. These types of foods are ideal for leaching out the minerals and nutrients for which a menopausal woman has the most need to conquer her symptoms. Nutrient deficiencies develop when the nutrients formerly supplied by the food itself are taken from body stores to handle the refined sugars that are eaten.

Don't think you can avoid the sugar problem by just staying with starches. Starches are chains of sugar molecules linked together by chemical bonds. When starches come in contact with digestive enzymes (starting in the mouth), they break down into, you guessed it, sugar.

Carbs also include the fiber foods, which are important for avoiding constipation. Fiber is also important in slowing the breakdown of starch to sugar, and refining removes fiber. This is why refined foods have a higher glycemic index than the same food unrefined—the fiber is less.

The glycemic index is only significant within the carbohydrate class, and though I question some of the numbers in the list, it's a good start. Fats and proteins don't stimulate insulin release, and that's what the index is all about—how fast the pancreas is stimulated to release insulin. There are, of course, foods with mixtures of carbs, protein, and fat. What's nice about some of these foods is that protein and fat also inhibit the rapid release of insulin, and subsequently a big blood sugar swing is avoided. An example of this effect is that of ice cream. Fat-free ice cream has a glycemic index of over 90, while the full-fat decadent stuff is rated at 69.[5]

PROTEINS

Proteins are organic amino acid-containing foods. They consist primarily of animal products (meat, fish, eggs, milk, cheese, etc.), but grains and legumes also contain protein, though it is the incomplete type (meaning not all 22 amino acids used in human nutrition are provided).

Protein is important stuff, as it has two main purposes. One is structural, for the formation of our bodies' organs, muscles, nerves, skin, and basically everything else. The other function is enzymatic, which is no less important. Enzymes are what permit most of the biochemical reactions in our bodies to take place at all. Hormones, antibodies, brain chemicals, you name it—complete protein better be there.

Complete is an important term, because if any of the 22 amino acids that make up the thousands of proteins our bodies produce are missing we can run into trouble. Vegans, or those who eat absolutely no animal products, are at the greatest risk for this, as the sulfur-containing amino acids are hard to obtain without any eggs or meat.

Unfortunately, high-protein foods can be expensive, so they can be slighted as a food class in favor of the refined carbs that are so prevalent in our modern civilization. If you evaluate value, however, protein substances take on a dimension worth every penny. They are heavier than carbs, and satisfy longer, not counting the fact that they do not stimulate the swings of insulin and blood sugar so prevalent with carbohydrate foods.

FATS

You may know most of these right off, but be careful because there are ones to avoid. Since my approach to handling your menopausal situation is a bit politically incorrect, you may be surprised at which ones you may eat on the plan.

Fats are, of course, a storage material for the body's energy fuel, but they do much, much more. For one, they are involved as the major component of the membrane of each cell in the body. Another important function of fats is that they serve as carriers for fat-soluble vitamins. The presence of fats is also required by body hormones. Clearly then, we need to think twice before trying to eliminate all fats from our diet.

What some people fail to realize is that all foods can convert to fat. Any carbohydrate or protein that isn't immediately burned can be readily stored as fat, so eating a diet with zero grams of fat means nothing. You can get plenty obese, and never eat a single gram of fat. Fun thought. I see it all the time, and I'll bet you have, too.

It is also important to realize that some fats are truly essential to humans because our bodies are unable to manufacture them from other fat molecules (fatty acids). These essential fatty acids (EFAs) come in two classes, omega-3 and omega-6, and need to be supplied in the diet. EFAs are polyunsaturated fats, meaning they are able to bond with hydrogen atoms. If polyunsaturated fats combine with hydrogen, they become more solid at room temperature. This is how vegetable oils (which are unsaturated) are made into margarine—by shooting hydrogen into them. Unfortunately, man-saturated fats like margarine have a slightly different structure than those made by nature, and this makes them undesirable (especially if you're trying to deal with menopausal symptoms.) Therefore we'll steer clear of both hydrogenated and partially-hydrogenated oils.

The need for EFAs is complicated by the fact that unsaturated oils are the ones that can go rancid. Saturated animal fats are immune from rancidity, basically because they are unable to take on extra hydrogen molecules. Fresh flax oil is my choice to supply the essential fatty acids we need. Fish oils, however, supply generous amounts of the omega-3 type, and certain vegetable oils, like primrose, borage, and black current, supply the omega-6 type. Flax oil is good for both; but it's important that it not go rancid, so it must be kept refrigerated and used quickly.

The point is, we want to avoid processed, adulterated, heated, rancid fats, staying with the freshest, most rancid-free fats as possible. That gives us one more factor on our side in handling the feel-bad, gain-weight thing we call menopause.

THE GOAL

To enable you to deal with the challenge of menopause, there are a few simple things that you can do:

- Avoid carbohydrates during the first week.
- Introduce carbohydrates gradually, starting the second week.
- Stay with unrefined, basically low glycemic-index foods when eating carbohydrates, always seeking nutrient density.
- Avoid processed, adulterated fats. (Animal fats *are* okay.)
- High quality proteins, as unprocessed as possible, need to be an important part of the routine.
- Eat combination whole foods (containing protein, fat, and carbs), such as fresh nuts and seeds.
- Throughout the entire process look for foods you introduce that make you feel worse or gain weight. These become your personal no-no's, to be avoided or used only rarely.

In most cases it is not necessary to be as strict as the Atkins diet in keeping carbohydrates out of the diet all the time. Also, the strict portions enforced by the zone-type diets are also not required, as long as you are alert to the problem presented by carbohydrates, introduce them slowly, and listen to your body when it tells you you've picked a bad one or eaten too much of one.

Supplement Use

I do not believe that, for most menopausal sufferers, successfully handling the situation with diet alone is possible. If it were, you probably wouldn't have had symptoms in the first place. Your reserves would have been sufficient to cover whatever cheating you've been doing. In fact, just for the record, I don't believe it's possible any longer, with the state of our food supply, for anyone to achieve anywhere near optimum health without nutritional supplements—no way.

Our diet is just not adequate anymore after all that we've done to it, even eating selectively. Bear in mind we're already starting with a woman known to have symptoms handling this phase of her life. It just usually takes more, though the proper foods make supplements more effective.

Things do wear out over time, or we'd all live forever. The machinery that helps us digest food, absorb nutrients, burn fat, stay well, repair damage, whatever, it all tends to lose efficiency over time. There are, in my opinion, dozens of supplements that can help the body's processes function better. However our purpose here is fairly singular, and the idea is offer some help without turning you into a major pill-popping health nut. (Maybe later.)

The bad news is that you likely will need some extra agents to obtain success. These will be listed in order of importance; then you can decide where to stop, or how much of each is needed to control the situation. Some people need very little. Others need the whole shooting match. The good news is that those agents exist.

MULTIVITAMIN/MINERAL SUPPLEMENT: To play the game you have to start with a whole team on the field, so I always start with a good multivitamin/multimineral supplement. There are many out there, as long as you're careful and read labels. Avoid those having 100 percent of the recommended daily allowance (RDA). These are more expensive for what you get, and just not strong enough. Stay with capsules and avoid time-release, so you know you'll actually absorb what you swallowed.

The minimum starter would be something like Solaray Multi-Energy, which is one capsule twice per day and available at most good health food stores. It can be purchased without iron, which I usually recommend. (Once a woman stops bleeding monthly, iron is just an additional stress on the body unless she is confirmed anemic by a doctor's determination.) There are other good ones, so compare labels, making sure that the calcium and magnesium content is more than just a few milligrams. My preference is for a supplement requiring six capsules per day, but some people may be unwilling to go that far, and I want everyone to succeed. It's possible with less, I just like to hedge my bets as much as possible. We'll be listing these options in the final section of this booklet.

VITAMIN C: I next add extra vitamin C. No multivitamins have enough to keep me happy, and the advantages go far beyond that of working with menopause. I usually recommend a minimum of 1000 milligrams twice per day, in capsule form.

DIGESTIVE ENZYMES: These are another important supplement. If weight gain has become a problem, but hadn't been earlier in life, I get very suspicious that the body is producing less than adequate amounts of digestive enzymes for adequately absorbing nutrients. This can be confirmed by expensive laboratory testing, but it seems easier to spend the money on supplements and find out that way. As nutrients from foods are better digested, discomfort symptoms also tend to be helped, but the weight situation tends to be the most graphic.

In selecting a good digestive enzyme, it is important to find one that contains enzymes to handle all three categories of foods (carbohydrates, fats, and proteins). These will be called amylolytic, lipolytic, and proteolytic, respectively, on the label. The most complete also include small amounts of a plant-based form of acid similar to stomach acid, called betaine hydrochloride. All good health food stores will have such products. Start with a half dose immediately after meals, then increase to full dose if there is no indigestion (uncommon). If any such symptoms occur, switch to any similar product that has all the listed enzymes at comparable strengths, but which omits betaine hydrochloride.

Introduce each supplement one at a time, one day apart, to make sure you don't have any sensitivity to a particular supplement. Lowering the dose for awhile, or changing brands, sometimes makes a difference. Once you begin taking these basic supplements, you'll have the starter team on your side. This, plus the food changes, may make all the difference you require (though I doubt it).

Now you can get specific, with nutrients that have a history of assisting with either menopausal pain symptoms or menopausal weight gain problems. Let's deal with discomfort first. No woman who has experienced hot flashes has much problem recognizing them. For the record, however, menopause can include an abundance of other neat symptoms, including irritability, night sweats, incontinence, sudden crying, strange sensations in the skin, headaches, and other less common goodies. There are improvements to be expected using dietary manipulation. Avoiding stimulants, smoking, and alcohol can be biggies, and sometimes laying off chocolate, hot drinks, and spicy foods can help. Often, however, more help is needed to establish real control over the symptomatic hassles of menopause.

COPING WITH MENOPAUSAL SYMPTOMS

To help cope with menopausal symptoms, add the following to your base plan of diet, multivitamin/mineral, C, and enzymes.

VITAMIN E (400-800 international units [IU]): Used for years in menopausal situations, it is known that requirements for this nutrient go up considerably at the time of menopause.[6] Nutritionally oriented practitioners have used it clinically for this problem since the 1930s, with published work by Drs. Wilfred and Evan Shute. Results usually take 2–3 weeks. Use a mixed tocopherol type, and if you can find a product with selenium included, that's even better.

BLACK COHOSH (*Cimicifuga racemosa*): This herb has an extensive history of benefiting menopausal symptoms, which includes clinical research.[7,8,9] Using a reputable brand, start with the recommended label dose.

DONG QUAI (*Angelica sinensis*): A long history of use, specifically for hot flashes.[10] Use as directed on the label.

CHASTE TREE BERRY (*Vitex agnus castus*): Use as directed on the label.

ESSENTIAL FATTY ACIDS: I have found that results are augmented with the addition of these nutrients that the body cannot manufacture. If you're into trying everything possible, add this. If cost is a factor, save this idea until you find the other recommendations to be inadequate. My preference is fresh flax oil, which contains both omega-6 and omega-3 classes. It is available in capsules, and I'd recommend 2-4 per day. However, some people prefer (and occasionally do better with) primrose, borage, or black currant oil, which contain primarily omega-6 acids only. Bear in mind that you must be taking the vitamin E first, as it protects against free radicals formed from the polyunsaturated nature of the oils.

Some combination of the above, along with the dietary changes, is usually effective. If not, natural hormone replacement (NHR) might be worth considering, which we'll discuss later. Bear in mind that this is *not* to be confused with hormone replacement therapy (HRT), or estrogen replacement therapy (ERT), so prominent in today's conventional medical care for menopausal women.

MENOPAUSAL WEIGHT GAIN

Now, just by cutting out the carbohydrates for a week, I have seen some stunning results concerning weight loss around menopause (plus at other times). This is not always the case, but it happens enough that I never cease to be amazed. Carbohydrate addiction, to me, is very real. When weight gain has not previously been a problem, only starting during menopause, dietary change alone seems to be more effective (though I still use digestive enzymes).

If this is the case with you, then you must decide when, and by how much, to reintroduce carbohydrates into your diet. Some people can add back as much as 40 percent unrefined carbs and continue to lose. Weight loss often ceases if you go beyond that point, even when it was working a bit below that point. If the carbs are of the refined, simple type, the switch back to weight gain tends to occur earlier.

Let's take the worst case scenario: nothing is working. You've been good on the diet (no carbs at all), taking your vitamins, and you haven't missed your digestive enzymes. Even should this have stopped further weight gain, if you aren't losing recently-acquired pounds, I then consider the plan a failure. At this point (should it be reached), other steps need to be considered. It can still be handled, so don't panic. There is still a lot left that you can do. The following supplements are additions to the base plan of diet, multivitamin/mineral, and enzymes, plus whatever is needed for menopausal symptoms.

L-CARNITINE (500 milligram capsules): This is an amino acid that is the only chemical in the body able to perform the final step in fat-burning, specifically the transporting of fatty acids in the bloodstream into the energy-producing units of our cells (mitochondria). Though not considered essential (our body can produce it from other amino acids), it is not uncommon for it to be undersupplied. Hence, supplementation can be very helpful, if not vital, as some people can even go into ketosis and still not burn the fat they have mobilized. The nutrient is taken as one, or preferably two, capsules twice a day *between* meals, using juice or water only.

LIPOTROPICS: These are a pair of water-soluble nutrients called choline and inositol, plus the amino acid methionine, and sometimes another compound called betaine. Backing up a step from the function of L-carnitine, the lipotropics are involved in the initial mobilization of fatty acids from their deposits as fat.[11,12] When I have had failures of diet and the general supplements alone, I first add the carnitine, and then the lipotropics, to the basic plan.

HYDROXYCITRIC ACID: This is a way to decrease appetite without the use of stimulants. HCA is derived from the herb *Garcinia cambogia*, and though it has an ancient history of appetite suppression and fat burning, there are now scientific studies in support of that.[13] This is my "icing on the cake," and it is often not necessary to go this far for results. However, it is a useful substance to enhance the weight loss process regardless of what other nutrients or carbohydrate level may be necessary. Really good producers of HCA don't just stop at the herb alone, and if you're going to do it, look for enhanced versions of the product. Its use is enhanced by the addition of small amounts of chromium, so I usually recommend supplements that include it with the HCA. The most comprehensive versions also add a substance called chitosan, an agent that binds fat and allows it to pass out of the system in the stool. (As this agent may adversely affect the body's level of beneficial bacteria over the long term, I only use this in the initial weight loss phase, if at all.)[14]

This whole routine avoids completely the class of weight loss agents called "thermogenic," which are known to be effective. These substances pump up the metabolism to help burn fat, and they do work. They even can be done safely, but if used as a "quick fix" you can get into trouble. They are not nutritional, and should be held for a last-ditch effort, as usually the above routine by itself allows for controlled loss.

For the record, if you add such agents to the menopause diet I put forward in this booklet, I'd recommend that you use the lowest dose possible, and stay below the "buzz" or "hyper" sensation that can come from taking stimulants like caffeine, ephedrine, adrenalin, theophylline, or combinations. Take them only 5 days out of every week, giving your adrenal glands a 2-day vacation, and add 200-500 mg of pantothenic acid as further protective nutritional insurance. I don't think they'll be necessary.

There are, however, a couple of other specific things you can do for occasional specific problems. You may find that digestive enzymes are inadequate at first, or possibly there is a residual feeling of indigestion. Should this occur, I recommend a short course of probiotics (acidophilus). This is a culture of "good guy" bacteria that we need by the billions in our intestines for proper digestion and other purposes. Look for capsules or powder types that contain billions of colony forming units (c.f.u.).

If you have trouble with carbohydrate cravings and just can't control them, you might try 250-500 of L-glutamine on an empty stomach. While in the early phase of trying to avoid carbohydrates, this may prove helpful.

There are reports of a newer agent, 5-HTP (5-hydroxytryptophan), that is helpful in curbing appetite and specifically carbohydrate cravings. This may be the case, as its precursor tryptophan helped in a similar way until it was made available by prescription only (for purely political purposes). Using 5-HTP raises serum levels (outside the cell) of serotonin, yet the body was meant to have high levels only within cells; therefore, I can't yet fully recommend it for any extended period.

Hormones

A real discussion of hormone therapy, and its use, is well beyond the scope of this little book. However, hormone therapy is so prevalent in the treatment of menopausal problems that we should at least touch on the subject.

We hope to be able to get the job done with diet, supplements, and herbs, thereby avoiding the use of any external hormones. I believe you have a real shot at that being the case. However, there may be times when such use may be necessary, at least temporarily (not to mention hormone use for osteoporosis). If such medications are considered, I strongly urge you to examine natural hormone replacement, not the use of today's synthetic (or non-natural) estrogen and progesterone replacements.

There's a lot of bad news concerning conventional hormone replacement therapy (HRT). It originally began as estrogen replacement therapy (ERT), but the use of unopposed estrogen (without progesterone) caused concern because of the incidence of endometrial cancer and blood clots. As a result, combined treatment with the two drugs was instituted (HRT).

The problem is, neither the estrogen nor the progesterone given to nearly all American women on hormones is chemically the same as the hormone of the same name occurring within a woman's body. These prescription drugs are altered, patented drugs that mimic parts of the real estrogen and progesterone molecules, but are different enough to cause some real trouble. Part of that includes the fact that synthetic progesterone (progestin) causes so many symptoms for women that most won't continue to take it. Estrogen also causes all sorts of symptoms.[15] Both synthetic classes are also dangerous.[16]

Did you know that real progesterone causes basically no symptoms, and carries all sorts of beneficial effects? What's more, when human estrogens (there are actually three, not just one) are given in the proper proportions, there is actually a protective effect on both endometrial and breast cancer.[17] But most "estrogen" that a woman receives by prescription fails to include all of three different types made by the body. The selection is for strength and patentability. Unfortunately, the woman's natural hormone that has a protective benefit against cancer (estriol) happens to be the weakest from a hormone standpoint, so it isn't normally used. The common form used today is Premarin, a name that comes from the drug's source: pregnant mare's urine. The bottom line is that you should know exactly what it is that you are putting into your body, and what its possible adverse effects can be.

This whole topic was brought to our attention by John R. Lee, M.D., a brilliant doctor from California who has been using natural progesterone to help with not only menopausal symptoms, but also osteoporosis, heart disease, fibrocystic breast disease, and more. He found that the easiest way to get estrogen is by using topical creams, either prescription (from a "compounding" pharmacist only) or at good health food stores. They even make incredible moisturizers. However, be careful to get creams that are already converted to actual progesterone. They nearly all come from the Mexican yam plant as a base source, but some are left in a form that must be converted to real progesterone, and the human body is not adept at doing that.

A superb, simple, inexpensive explanation of natural hormone replacement (both estrogen and progesterone) is available in the book *Natural Hormone Replacement*, by Jonathan Wright, M.D. If your health food store doesn't have it, you can call 1-800-543-3873 to order a copy. Any of the works of John R. Lee, M.D., are also a wonderful education.

The goal is to allow you to lose weight and avoid menopausal symptoms as naturally as possible, avoiding the use of prescription medication. I think you have a good shot at it. My suggestion would be to give the plan a one or two month trial. If, at that point, you feel the benefits are just not enough, then you at least have an option that carries far fewer side effects and dangers than the current medications in conventional prominence. If you then decide that hormone therapy is necessary as an addition, look for a doctor who will use or monitor natural hormone therapies. You may even need additional doses of other hormones, depending on your bloodwork.

Exercise

I'm not an exercise freak. I don't believe massive amounts are really necessary to get the job of living life done. This may be somewhat reassuring at a time when the last thing you feel like doing is running a marathon. However, for the total couch potato experiencing menopausal hot flashes there is some bad news: exercise helps them go away. In a study of hundreds of menopausal women, none of whom took hormones, it was found that 3.5 or more hours per week of regular exercise made for milder, less frequent hot flashes.[18] If you can get yourself to consider some mild to moderate exercise, it is highly recommended.

The ideal plan is to find something you like to do. If you're a tennis fanatic or bodybuilding nut, then exercise is not a problem. It's those who really don't enjoy any particular form of exercise that I'm talking to right now. (All others can skip ahead to the next section and start the plan.)

If you are not an exerciser, my goal here is to get you doing *something*. It isn't necessary to measure target heart rates or be particularly aerobic.

The idea is to increase circulation, and almost any exertion can do that, so there's no need to feel like you're missing out on some therapeutic benefit because you just can't force yourself to get up at five in the morning to get a big workout in.

There are simple things you can do, and anything that does any toning at all helps our goal. Increased blood flow helps distribute nutrients more efficiently, and assists in the removal of cellular waste products. The list gets longer; exercise has lots of advantages. So, for the non-athlete, how do you do that without going nuts?

One of the best things you can do for your body is to stretch. Slowly twist left and right, turn your head in all directions, circle your arms, and begin the effort for toe-touches (the operative word is *slowly*).

Another suggestion is, first thing in the morning, before you get up, to throw the pillow down over your feet, slide down in the bed, and do a few sit-ups. At that moment of the day, it's likely no less desirable than actually getting up. Do a few, and see if you can do a few more tomorrow. It even makes getting up easier.

If you like hitting things, but chasing tennis balls around the parking lot isn't your idea of a good time, consider badminton. It's easier to learn than tennis, not as high output as racquetball, inexpensive, and great exercise. Running, even jogging, isn't necessary. Brisk walking is wonderful, low impact (avoid concrete), and needs a minimum of equipment.

Now, here's my favorite: buy a mini-trampoline. These are small, about three feet in diameter, with springs or bungee cords, and stand on short legs. Some even have folding legs, so the device can be slipped under a bed once you're finished. It's a form of exercise that has everything going for it. It's an indoor sport, it's incredible for increasing circulation, and it's fun. It can be done rain or shine, nobody has to watch you do it, and you can vary the intensity easily.

My recommendation, for those who hate exercise, is to try light bouncing on the trampoline during a TV show. It takes no additional time at all, and you can bounce as much or as little as desired, all the while getting benefit. Once you get tired of bouncing, just stay there a few minutes rocking up and down on the balls of your feet. That alone assists blood flow. If, in a few minutes, you feel you can bounce a little more, your exercise machine is right there under your feet.

Whatever you do, try to do some form of light exercise; something that raises your heart rate, but not to the point of pain or exhaustion. Check with your doctor to see what he feels is acceptable for whatever medical situation may apply to you, and give it a go. The results might pleasantly surprise you.

The Weight-Loss Plan

You've been introduced to the principles of this routine for losing weight and controlling symptoms during the menopausal years. Since there are two goals, and some may not need them both, you may incorporate what parts of the plan fit you the best, and tailor what techniques work best for you. Everyone is unique, so a concrete plan for everyone is essentially a pipe dream.

My recommendation is to be as compliant as possible during the first one to two weeks. This is when the diet is the strictest, and the rules are the least fun. It doesn't last that long. Then, any changes you make are toward a less strict regimen. Bear in mind that, though individual meals are not prescribed, undesirable foods are pretty clear, especially during the first two weeks. Try to be good. Seeing results often doesn't take that long.

Nutrients and herbs are listed in order of my personal preference, which doesn't have a big scientific ring to it. Here again, I'm leaning on experience, both mine and others, to establish what gives you the best chance at improvement. Something down the list may actually be the best answer for you personally. I also recommend stricter than average compliance to low glycemic index ranges. I figure you'll give this plan one try, and I want it to have the best chance to succeed.

Once you feel better, at that point you can taper any supplements you are taking down to the lowest dose that continues to get the job done, and try higher glycemic foods. That's it! The very best of luck to you in your efforts to attain a healthy state. You are *not* over the hill, and you shouldn't feel that way.

Dietary Rules

GENERAL

1. Eat slowly and chew thoroughly. This is no joke, and its importance cannot be overemphasized.
2. Take a short break mid-meal; quit eating if/when satisfied.
3. Drink plenty of good water. Spring is preferred; no city water. Don't go crazy, as it's not necessary to get sick drinking tons of the stuff. Drink until your thirst is gone, maybe just a little more, and that's it.
4. Eat frequently, before you're starving, at which point you lose all willpower.

WEEK 1

1. Avoid all carbohydrates, simple or complex. This includes fruits and their juices, flour, pasta, breads, and most vegetables and/or their juices. Acceptable foods during this period are included in Table 1 below. Basically, all high-protein foods are allowed, and fat is not a big consideration (unless you do something weird like go on a whipped cream diet or something).

2. The allowable carbohydrates are selected due to the fact that they have minimal glycemic influence.

3. If you require more regimentation, any good high-protein, very low-carbohydrate diet is fine for the first week. *The Atkins Diet Revolution*, by Robert Atkins, M.D., is still the best, though you normally will end up with more carbohydrates at the end (maintenance) than with his diet, more nearly approaching the 40 percent carbohydrate zone-type diets. These are *The Zone*, by Barry Sears, Ph.D., or *40-30-30 Fat Burning Nutrition*, by Joyce and Gene Daoust (do not use this book's glycemic index).

All **meats** allowed (without added fillers, coatings, MSG, sugars, starches; avoid nitrates/nitrites);
All **fish**;
All **fowl**;
All **shellfish**;
Eggs, fertile preferred (try to prepare in ways that do not break the yolk while cooking);
Green leafy vegetables: head lettuce, romaine, parsley, spinach, collard greens, beet tops, kale;
Salad vegetables: celery, cucumber, radish, pepper (green/ red);
Cabbage, sauerkraut;
Garlic;
Bamboo shoots;
***Onions**;
***String beans**;
***Squash**;
***Broccoli, cauliflower, Brussels sprouts**;
***Asparagus**;
***Avocado**;
***Turnips**;
***Okra**;
***Pumpkin**;
***Water Chestnuts**;
***Cheese**, if not sensitive to dairy; use stronger ones like brie, parmesan, etc., so you can use smaller amounts, and save cottage cheese for week two, as it is higher in carbohydrates;
***Artificial sweeteners** as needed; Stevia (the best choice)- this is an herb that is extremely sweet, available in health food stores as extract or powder; use as desired.

(*Note: with any of the items marked with an asterisk, you need to start with small servings to see how you tolerate them)

NOT ALLOWED IN FIRST WEEK: beans (other than green, string, waxed); potatoes (any type); sweet pickles; peas; corn; cashews; milk (heavy cream is permitted); no fruit; no alcohol; *nothing* with sugar or starch (including flour/flour products, pasta, breads of any type, coatings, fillings, etc.). Be conscientious here, and you save hassles later.

TABLE 1: FOODS FOR WEEK 1

WEEK 2 AND ON

1. Using the lowest possible numbers in the Glycemic Index as a basic guide, you introduce desired carbohydrate-containing foods *one at a time,* never more than one per day, preferably every other day. Look for any symptoms that are uncomfortable. They may be runny nose, irritability, congestion, cramping, headache, fatigue, or anything else. Make sure the food is not responsible for the adverse effects before adding it to your routine permanently. If you run into a problem, back up to the previous status and begin again.
2. Nuts and seeds are very low on the index, and tend to be good items to introduce next, while still maintaining decent weight loss. Caution with cashews (more carbohydrates).
3. Cottage cheese is okay to test here.
4. The index has starred items. These are foods that should be used minimally, even though their ranking in the list may or may not be favorable. These items have low nutrient density, which is important to to avoid as much as possible for success in either the weight-loss or the symptom control endeavor.
5. Bear in mind that there are variations in the Glycemic Index, depending on the labs doing the testing, the quality of the foods tested, and of course the human subjects involved. Not all whole wheat flour is exactly alike, for example, as soil nutrition, fiber and fat content, and other factors can vary. You can also find indexes that list the same food, both refined and unrefined, as having the same glycemic rating. I find this hard to explain, as fat content, protein content, and fiber content are the factors that determine how high the number is. I ignore indexes that show refined and unrefined foods as having the same index ranking.
6. Some indexes use white flour as a ranking of 100. We don't use that system, preferring the one that uses glucose as a value of 100. This leaves only maltose with a` higher ranking (110). If you find a "white flour=100" list you can do an approximate conversion to a "glucose=100" list by multiplying the numbers by 0.7.
7. The slower you introduce new foods, the better you will become aware of their effects on your goals.

Table 2 (on following page) is a general guide consolidated from several lists; thus, accuracy varies. And as in Table 1, for items marked with an asterisk, you must start with small portions to see how you tolerate them.)

BEANS
baby lima 32; baked 43; black 30; brown 38; butter beans 31; chickpeas 33; kidney 27-43; navy 38; pinto 42; red lentils 27-38; split peas 32; soy 18; garbanzo 30

BREADS
*bagel 72; *Kaiser roll 73; pita 57; pumpernickel 49; *rye 64; rye, whole 42-50; *white 72; whole wheat 50; *half bread 65; *waffles 76

CEREALS
All Bran 44; Bran Chex 58; *Cheerios 74; *Corn Bran 75; *Corn Chex 83; *Cornflakes 83; *Cream of Wheat 66; *Crispix 87; Grapenuts 67; *Grapenuts Flakes 80; *Life 66; Muesli 60; *NutriGrain 66; Oatmeal 53; *Oatmeal (instant) 66; *Puffed Wheat 74; Rice Bran 19; *Rice Chex 89; *Rice Krispies 82; Shredded Wheat 69; *Special K 54; Muesli 60; *Total 76

COOKIES/CRACKERS
oatmeal 55; *shortbread 64; *vanilla wafers 77; *Kavli Norwegian 71; *rye 63; *saltine 72

DESSERTS
*angel food cake 67; bran muffin 60; *danish 59; fruit bread 47; *pound cake 54; *sponge cake 46

FRUIT
apple [w/skin] 38; *apricot, canned 64; apricot, dried 30; banana 61; banana, unripe 30; cherries 22; *fruit cocktail 55 [no sugar]; grapefruit 25; *grapes 45; kiwi 52; mango 55; orange 43; *orange juice 49; pear 36; *pineapple 66; plum 24; *raisins 64; strawberries 32; watermelon 72 [nutrient-dense juice]

GRAINS
barley 22; buckwheat 54; bulgur 47; chickpeas 36; *cornmeal 68; *hominy 40; millet 75; *rice, instant 91; *rice, white 70-88; rice, whole (brown) 50-59; rye 34 [whole only]; sweet corn 55-70; *popcorn 85; whole wheat 41

JUICES
*apple 41; grapefruit 48; *orange 57; *pineapple 46.

MILK PRODUCTS
*chocolate milk 34; *ice cream 50-69; ice cream, fat-free 90+; milk 34 [the more fat the lower the glycemic rating]; yogurt 38 [no sugar, use stevia or artificial if must]

NUTS
almonds 15; pecans 15; peanuts 15; walnuts 15;

PASTA
linguine, durum 50; *macaroni & cheese 64; *white 50-67; whole wheat 40-42;

SUGARS
*maltose 110; *glucose 100; *fructose [not acceptable, even with ranking, due to other damage to body] 20; *table sugar, cane or beet (avoid) 59-83; *honey 90

VEGETABLES
beet 65; green veggies, tomatoes, lemon, mushrooms <15; *baked potatoes 95 [may scoop out and eat skin with some of the potato and butter/sour cream to lower rating]; *mashed potatoes 90; carrots 85; peas 50 (frozen may be higher); *boiled potatoes 70; corn 55-70 [caution here]

TABLE 2: FOODS FOR WEEK 2 AND ON
(GLYCEMIC INDEX)

Supplements

GENERAL

Multivitamin (minimum strength), 25 mg of each major B-vitamin (B6, B2, B6), while 50 mg of each is preferred; capsules taken twice per day or even six times per day are usually better. Avoid time release and avoid added iron where possible, unless confirmed anemic.
Vitamin C, 1000 mg/cap, 1 twice/day (ascorbate form if needed due to any gastric upset).
Digestive enzymes, full-spectrum type, taken immediately after meals.

FOR WEIGHT LOSS (add to above if necessary):

L-carnitine, 500 mg/cap, 1-2 twice/day between meals, water/juice only.
Lipotropics (choline, inositol, methionine combined), max dose, twice/day.
HCA (hydroxycitric acid), as Citrichrome, Citrimax, or equivalent, twice/day. (The added chromium and chitosan are helpful.)

FOR SYMPTOMS (add as needed):

Vitamin E (mixed tocopherols), 400-800 iu/day, with selenium, if possible.
Black cohosh, maximum dose recommended on label.
Dong quai, maximum dose recommended on label.
Chaste tree berry, maximum dose recommended on label.
(Flaxseed oil capsules, 2-4/day, optional.)
(Real progesterone cream, as needed, daily for 3 weeks of every month.)

FOR ADDITIONAL HELP (add as needed)

Probiotics (acidophilus), before meals and bedtime, for digestive difficulties.
L-glutamine, 500 mg between meals, for carbohydrate cravings.
5-HTP, as directed on label, possibly helpful for carbohydrate cravings.

References

1. NRC RDA recommendations for enrichment.
2. Guyten, A.C., *Textbook of Medical Physiology*, W.B. Saunders Co. Phil, PA, 1976.
3. The many works of Robt. Atkins,MD.
4. The best source of information on the low fat controversy, impeccably documented, is available from the Price-Pottenger Nutrition Foundation, 1-800-FOODS-4-U.
5. *40-30-30 Fat Burning Nutrition*, pp. 35-36.
6. Davis, A., *Let's Eat Right to Keep Fit*, HBJ, '70,pp 150-1.
7. *Nutrition & Healing*, Wright, J.V., Gaby, A.R., June, '96,p.2, 10.
8. Duker, E.M., et al. Effects of extracts from *Cimicifuga racemosa* on gonadotrophin release in menopausal women and ovariectomized rats. *Planta Medica* 57:4420-424, '91.
9. *Health & Nutrition Breakthroughs*, Nov., '97,pp 32-34.
10. Royal, P., *Herbally Yours*, Sound Nutrition, '82, p 84.
11. *Vitamin Bible*, Mindell, E.,1979,pp 174-178.
12. "Lipotropics," article by Mindell, E., Ph.D., 1980.
13. *Pocket Herbal Reference*, Elkins, R., M.H., 1997, pp 43-44.
14. Tanaka, Y., et al, Chitin, 'Biomaterials; 4/97, 18(8):591-5.
15. *Monthly Prescribing Reference*, May,'98,pp.118-122.
16. Ibid.
17. Wright, J. et al, *Natural Hormone Replacement*, Smart Pub.,'97.
18. Hammer, M.,et al. "Does physical exercise influence freq. of postmen. hot flushes?" *Acta Ob/Gyn Scand.*, 69:409-412,1990.